The Chakra Healing Collection

Energy Healing Super Set

Daniel Amos

I0427962

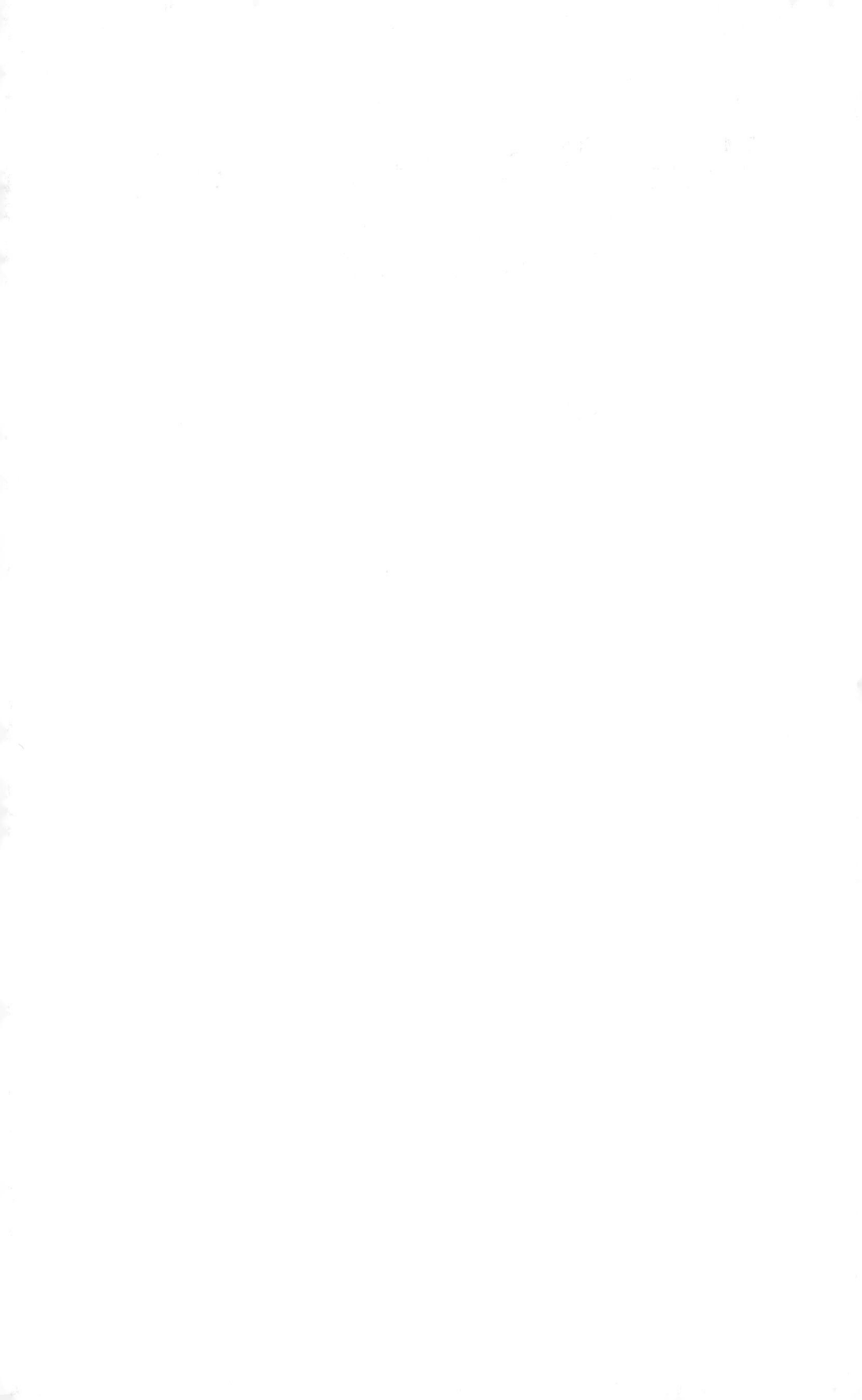

TABLE OF CONTENTS

THE CHAKRA CODE
How Balancing the 7 Chakras Will Bring You Instant Health, Wealth, and Happiness

Introduction

I want to thank you and congratulate you for downloading the book, The Chakra Code.

This book contains proven steps and strategies on how to help you balance the energy centers of your body, known as the chakras, and thus bring your emotional, physical, and spiritual life back into balance.

Over the next few chapters, I will be showing you what the chakras are and how to interact with them. Over the course of this little guide, we will look at the sort of activities, colors, exercises, and foods that will help you clear each energy center and feel more capable, healthier, and more confident about yourself!

Thanks again for purchasing this book, and I hope you enjoy it!

CHAPTER 1: WHAT ARE THE CHAKRAS

The term 'chakra' itself is ancient Sanskrit for wheel and refers to the spinning nature of the energy centers that are situated throughout the body. This is also called energy medicine, or energetic therapy, and is based on ancient spiritual teachings from India, China, and Japan.

The ancient physicians and healers of these areas were aware of something called the subtle body, or the energy that flows in and around our body, which is attracted to certain areas and helps our organs to function properly. Chinese medicine calls the pathways that this energy takes the **meridians**, and their alternative therapies of **acupuncture** and **Chinese herbal therapy** depend upon it.

These meridians take the energy from part of the body to the next, literally through hundreds of chakra points (usually near or over glands, nerve clusters and major organs). However, there are seven places around the body where all of these meridians meet up and form the major chakras, the ones that regulate the whole body and not just small areas.

These main energy centers take in energy from our environment in an active and a passive way. They take in energy not only from sunlight, from fresh air, and from the rhythms of night and day but also from the food that we eat and from our habits and routines. If we are healthy, then the meridians flow easily and the chakras are in constant state of health. Their natural state is to be spinning, churning, recycling, and renewing the energy, like the pulmonary blood systems.

For reasons that we will describe below, it has long been believed that particular chakras are regulating particular emotional habits and states of being as well. In effect, by balancing your chakras, you can make a positive and immediate effect upon your confidence, health, and success.

The Mind–Body Unity

Have you noticed that when you are hungry, you are also more likely to be irritable?

Have you noticed that when you are stressed, sad, or depressed, you are much more likely to get physically ill?

Just as Western science is only now coming to understand that the mind and the body are inseparable, so Eastern science has always known that the mind and the body are one unit. What you think and feel affect the body, and vice versa: how you act, what you eat, and what you do to occupy your time affect your emotions, your thought patterns, and ultimately your confidence and efficiency.

The ancients believed that it was because of this subtle body that the two – the mind and the body – were intertwined. The energy was called *chi, qi,* or *prana* in various traditions and was thought to be the lifeblood of the universe. In today's world, we can just as easily understand it as subatomic vibration, or pure energy transfer, which we know all material and seemingly immaterial atoms and particles are made of.

The chakras work as connectors between the mind and the body and can be understood as the energetic 'organs' of this subtle body. If you are experiencing physical problems or ailments, then there is quite a good likelihood that there will be an energetic imbalance somewhere. You may be being afflicted with negative emotions and low self-worth or have deep, unresolved issues that you need to balance.

By working directly with the chakras, we can target these feelings and beliefs and bring this subtle and physical body into a healthy whole.

How Can We Diagnose a Chakra Imbalance?

Chakras are the spinning circles of our energy system, pulling energy in that needs to be renewed and transmitting healthier energy outwards once again. They are located vertically along the center line of the body, over the spine. Each one is associated with an endocrine center of the body and so regulates the flow of hormones, energy, and stimulation in that area.

If they stop to work correctly and become blocked or imbalanced, then they will either pull in too much energy or even cease to work completely. This has a knock-on effect on the rest of the other chakras, and so secondary and associated systems can occur.

If we have problems in any of the following areas of the body where the chakras are located, then we can immediately presume chakra imbalance:

Root troubles: IBS; stomach upset; and difficulty in sitting, sleeping, or lying down

Sacral troubles: sexual health, digestion, and fertility problems

Solar plexus troubles: sense of unease, low self-worth, and anxiety

Heart troubles: arrhythmia; low or high blood pressure; sadness; and unable to feel dynamic, energized, or happy

Throat troubles: problem in breathing, coughs, difficulty in talking, colds, and sinus problems.

Third eye troubles: insight, vision, and eyesight problems and paranoia

Crown chakra troubles: thinking problems, foggy minded, and daydreaming

Assessing Chakra Health

Luckily, as well as assessing ourselves using the above list of symptoms, there is also a very easy way to diagnose chakra imbalances.

You will need only

a pendulum

Using a crystal, stone, or favorite dowsing object on some thin twine, you can hold the pendulum over each chakra and 'ask' for its size, speed, and direction. Using this simple method, you can assess each one to see if some are spinning fast or too slow and are over large or too small.

Place the pendulum over each chakra, asking your questions as to its condition and state, and try to detect whether you feel any residue of heat, cold, unease, or sickness.

You can also use the same technique to ask which stone, crystal, color, or medicine to use for each chakra, by holding the pendulum over each and asking for the results!

Tools to Balance the Chakras

Finally, there are a lot of tools available out there to balance the chakras, and you can use any one or a combination of these listed below to help you become healthier, balanced, and more confident:

Color therapy

Crystals

Reiki

Meditation and visualizations

Diet

Yoga

Positive thinking and affirmations

Physical exercise

Aromatherapy

CHAPTER 2: CHAKRA GUIDE

Listed below is a guide to all of the main chakras of the body, including what they are associated with. You can also use this list to help you diagnose any particular problems that you might have with a particular chakra imbalance.

Root Chakra

Located at the base of the spine and tailbone area, the chakra sits underneath the spine and the body. Represents our foundation and our feelings of being grounded. Associated with security, basic living needs, and survival issues.

Sacral Chakra

Located in the lower abdomen, about 2–3 inches below our navel. Represents our connection to others and willingness to accept new experiences, pleasure, and feeling satisfied.

Solar Plexus Chakra

Located in the upper abdomen, just under the rib cage. Represents our feelings of abundance and confidence.

Heart Chakra

Located in the center of our chest, right above our heart, the heart chakra represents our feelings of love, joy, and peace.

Throat Chakra

Located in the center of the throat, the throat chakra represents our ability to communicate, our self-expression, our confidence, and our awareness of the truth.

Third Eye Chakra

Located in the center of the forehead between the eyes, the third eye chakra represents our intuition, imagination, wisdom, and ability to think and to make decisions.

Crown Chakra

The highest chakra in the body; the crown chakra is located at the very top of the head, as if above the line of the spine. It represents our connection to spirituality, wisdom, and bliss.

CHAPTER 3: HEALING THE CHAKRAS WITH LIGHT

Chakras and Light

An important part of chakra balancing is working with light and visualization. This can be done through merely visualizing the light entering certain chakras in your body, as a form of meditation, or you can use actual color therapy, such as different colored lamps or wearing different colored clothes to surround yourself with that energy.

The reason that the chakras respond so well to color therapy is that, of all of the balancing techniques, colors are the closes to pure energy. As we all know, the purest form of light is that coming from the sun, moons, and stars. To be at our most natural, we must make sure that we are exposed often to this source of light. As we ourselves are beings of energy in its heaviest, material form, we can restore ourselves to this purer vibration by using the colors of the spectrum to align our chakras.

Each chakra you will see has its own color associated with it, and by choosing to surround or to mentally encourage certain colors, you will be literally 'feeding' or protecting that chakra.

Different Ways to Use Color Therapy

Wear the chosen color in your outer garments.

Wear or wrap a scarf of the chosen color around the chosen chakra.

Lying down, lay a light scarf or other light material of your chosen color over the chakra, meditate, and relax.

Mentally visualize yourself being bathed in the chosen color.

Carry a crystal colored by your chosen color, and, during the day, set it in front of you and turn it towards you. Imagine it beaming that color straight into your subtle body!

The Different Healing Chakra Colors

White diamond – Used for the crown chakra, this is an almost blinding, purifying light that energizes you and raises your energetic level to higher spiritual planes.

Emerald green flame – This is a healing, physically nourishing viridian light, used to heal the heart chakra and lower.

Violet flame – Associated with sacral chakra and all chakras in the body under the neck; represents the divine masculine and the divine feminine unifying together to heal your emotions and heart.

Rose pink light – Most clearly associated with the sacral and the base chakras, the rose pink light infuses your aura with the unconditional feeling of safety and protection, making it excellent for inner child healing.

Sunshine yellow – Associated with our sacral, solar plexus, and heart chakras; represents Christ consciousness or charity, goodwill, and generosity.

Gold light –A much stronger version of the sunshine yellow ray; this color is associated instead with the whole body and each chakra and is good for generating peace, decreasing stress, and achieving harmony. This is excellent to end with after heavy energy work.

CHAPTER 4: HEALING THE FIRST CHAKRA

Otherwise known as the Kundalini, root, or base chakra, the base chakra is symbolized by fire and the snake or dragon. It is the physical and emotional foundation of the body itself, as it is situated under the tailbone and at the end of the spine. The root chakra stimulates the vital forces throughout the body like digestion, energy, and hunger and assists us to feel grounded, physical, and 'real.'

The most important thing that we can associate with the root chakra is the fight or flight response, as it is tightly concerned with our most basic survival issues. In the modern world, this can also translate as our financial security, worries or anxieties relating to our home, our sensation of belonging, and our connection to our family.

Glandular system: Adrenal glands

Incense: Cedar wood

Musical note: Middle C

Vowel sound: U (pronounced you)

Element: Earth or rock

Crystals: Agate, garnet, ruby, bloodstone, jasper, and hematite

Color: Red

Healing exercises:

Practice Kundalini yoga to strengthen and awaken this chakra and lower spine.

Stomping and dancing bare feet on the ground. This chakra is all about feeling grounded, physical, and secure.

Healing foods:

Anything red colored (apples, beets, and tomatoes)

Spices such as tabasco and cayenne!

Earth vegetables and tubers

Red meat and animal protein

CHAPTER 5: HEALING THE SECOND CHAKRA

The second or sacral chakra is otherwise known as spleen, sexual, or Svadhisthana chakra and represents our sexuality, our feelings of satisfaction, and our emotions, but is not merely limited to our love life! As the wellspring of dynamic creativity, the second chakra is also the source of our creativity and inspiration, especially when linked to emotional enthusiasm, the flush of new relationships, and the ability to connect to others in a new way. When the chakra is functioning correctly, it encourages us to be able to maintain healthy relationships, to enjoy ourselves, and to let go of emotions when we no longer feel them.

However, when this chakra is not working correctly, it leads to physical complications in the bladder, spleen, kidneys, and the sexual organs as well as emotional problems such as jealousy, guilt, and obsession. Essentially, these lower-abdomen organs are all about purification and enjoyment, and so this chakra is about our ability to partake in life as well as to move on.

Related incense: Damiana, gardenia, and orris root

Related glandular system: Sexual

Musical note: D

Related sound: 'O' (as in 'home')

Related herbs: Coriander and fennel

Element: Water

Crystals: Amber, citrine, gold topaz, moonstone, calcite, gold, coral, and carnelian.

Color: Orange

Healing exercises:

Pelvic thrusts

Yoga (cobra pose)

Healing foods:

Anything orange colored, such as oranges, tangerines, and clementines

Lightly spiced foods, nuts, and seeds

CHAPTER 6: HEALING THE THIRD CHAKRA

The third, solar plexus or Manipura, chakra is located at the base of the rib cage and at the top of the abdomen and is represented by the color yellow. This chakra is often associated with birds and flight, as it is the first chakra that really helps us to travel outside of our astral body and connect with others, places, and things. Physically, this chakra is associated with the musculature system, the stomach, our general metabolic rate, and our nervous system.

To understand the third chakra, we need to understand that it sits atop the other two, more fundamental, 'survival' chakras that are essentially about yourself. The third chakra is the first chakra that is about self-acceptance, confidence, and our ability to connect with others. It is a step away from the selfishness of pleasure and survival issues and towards community and friendship.

When the third chakra is well organized, we feel comfortable with our ability to reach out and connect with others and are able to organize oneself well and ably. When this chakra is blocked or imbalanced, then it leads to profound problems with our ability to work in a team or to function well in any group situation. This can manifest as a difficulty dealing with hierarchy, an inability to make friends, anger, and frustration.

Essentially, this chakra will regulate our self-esteem and self-confidence as a social being. If we feel unhappy or frustrated about ourselves, then that naturally leads to our diminished capacity to relate to others and therefore develop resentment.

Related incense: Marigold, cinnamon, and carnation

Related herbs: Lemon balm and goldenseal

Related glandular system: The gallbladder, liver, and spleen

Musical note: E

Chakra sound: 'O' as in top, pop, or dollop

Element: Fire

Healing crystals: Gold topaz, tiger eye, amber, gold calcite, pure gold, and citrine

Color: Yellow

Healing exercises:

Kundalini yoga (especially the boat pose)

Dancing and shaking (especially movement of the hips)

Healing foods:

Anything yellow colored, such as corn, split peas, and some beans

Grains and fiber such as whole wheat, granola, or whole grain

Light herbal teas, particularly peppermint and mint

CHAPTER 7: HEALING THE FOURTH CHAKRA

The fourth, heart or Anahata, chakra is located right in the center of the chest, around the area (and just above) of the heart. It is represented by mammals and human life and is associated with our emotional heart and our feelings. You will have noticed by now that all of the lower chakras relate to the self in one form or another, either our most primitive feelings and associations; moving on towards our feelings of self-satisfaction, personal fulfillment, and confidence; or now towards others in the truest sense: that of affection and compassion.

Our fourth chakra influences how we relate to others and other beings in the world, whether through joy and acceptance or through pain and fear. As such, it dictates our connection to nature, to the plant world, and to our families and others. It is the heart chakra where the famous 'Christ energy' or our unconditional acceptance and joy in others arise. Emotions associated with this chakra are compassion, love, forgiveness, empathy, trust, our sense of emotional equilibrium, and being at ease with life. If we have a strong heart chakra, then we may feel a strong calling towards humanitarian ends.

If the heart chakra is out of balanced or maligned, then we may physically suffer from respiratory or lung problems, as well as heart burn or other disorders of the cardiovascular system. The most obvious symptom of problems with this chakra is, however, emotional heartache, depression, and feelings of pervasive emptiness. Any sort of problems to do with love, such as feelings of being unloved, unworthy, or being emotionally unstable, are due to this chakra.

Related incense: Lavender, yarrow, orris root, jasmine, meadowsweet, and marjoram

Associated herbs: Rue and saffron

Related glandular system: Thymus

Musical note: F

Chakra sound: 'A' as in far, far, and car

Element: Air

Crystals: Green jade, green aventurine, emerald, malachite, fluorite, ruby, moldavite, kunzite, rose quartz, chrysoprase, and pink tourmaline

Color: Green or gold

Healing exercises:

Bikram yoga

Sufi heart exercises (accepting and generating love)

Sun salutation (yoga)

CHAPTER 8: HEALING THE FIFTH CHAKRA

The fifth, throat or Vishuddha, chakra is symbolized by the element of ether, purity, and the human race. It represents artistic expression, our ability to speak the truth and to communicate, dream, and our good judgment. Physically, it is located for men behind the Adam's apple, and for women, in the center of the throat. It is physically associated with all instances of the teeth, mouth, throat, and thyroid glands.

As the chakra of essential communication, the fifth chakra is connected to our ability to travel out of our body – ranging from our speech that touches another's life, to dreaming, to out of body experiences, to clairaudience. When the fifth chakra is balanced and operating as it should, then it helps us to feel centered, happy, and responsible.

If, however, the fifth chakra is not working as it should, then this can express itself in the form of sore throats, throat infections, losing one's voice, earaches, and any problem associated with communication. Persistent problems with this chakra manifest as thyroid and sinus problems physically and a general level of exhaustion and being rundown – in very extreme cases, this equals chronic fatigue and fibromyalgia.

Emotionally, chronic problems with this chakra will lead to us being easily dominated by others and unable to 'find out own voice.'

Related incense: Benzoin and frankincense

Related herbs: Eugenia, vervain, and cloves

Associated glandular system: Thyroid

Musical note: G

Chakra sound: 'E' short, as in let, get, and bet

Element: Ether and earth

Color: Blue

Crystals: Blue sapphire, celestite, blue topaz, sodalite, lapis lazuli, aquamarine, azurite, kyanite, chalcedony, turquoise, and chrysocolla

Healing exercise:

Any sort of singing or chanting

Shoulder stands

Healing foods:

Fruit juices (any kind thereof)

Juices and teas

CHAPTER 9: HEALING THE SIXTH CHAKRA

The sixth, third eye or Ajna, chakra is situated in between the eyebrows and up an inch, most clearly associated with the notion of the third eye in parapsychology and mysticism. The sixth chakra represents our wisdom and insight and the element of the inquiring mind. Insight, even to the point of foresight, is its key attribute and as such represents how aware and alert we are mentally.

When this chakra is balanced, it allows us to peer deeply into the root causes of things and to develop our powers of intuition, not our 'gut instincts' but rather our powers of sixth sense, to be able to think laterally and to make correct deductions about people and situations that we encounter. To others, this well-developed and healthy sixth chakra will appear to verge on the paranormal, and for good reason, this chakra is the gateway chakra to the higher spiritual realms and helps to define our relationship to fantasy and reality. If the sixth chakra is spinning too fast, and it is larger than the rest of the chakras below, then the sufferer will become too occupied with fantasy, with others, thoughts, and the astral realms, leaving them feeling paranoid, afraid, or afflicted.

Symptoms of problems with this chakra are brain fog, poor attention spans, nightmares, and headaches, as well as general inability to be insightful or aware of others around us. Unlike the other chakras, the major problem with the sixth chakra is not if it is blocked but rather if it is open too early or too much. In chakra balancing, you will become aware that the chakras are interlinked and that they all build upon each other in a gradual and progressive way. When you are feeling safe and secure, then you are allowed to develop your relationship to pleasure and satisfaction. When you can look after yourself and your needs, then you are taught how to communicate and relate to others. This process is the process of each chakra opening up and developing in their natural order and occurs throughout our life and especially through our first 29 years.

If the sixth chakra opens or develops too early (such as with an obsessive preoccupation with daydreaming or fantasy and drugs or psychic practices), then the problem is not that it hasn't opened but that it is letting in too many messages about the astral and subtle realms and that the rest of our chakras and our mind–body unity cannot synthesize as yet, because they themselves haven't developed fully enough yet.

Related incense: Star anise, mugwort, saffron, and acacia

Related herbs: Sandalwood

Related aromatherapy: Lavender, rosemary, and gardenia

Related glandular system: Pituitary

Musical note: A

Chakra sound: 'A' as in me and sea

Element: Water and light

Color: Royal purple and indigo

Crystals: Fluorite, azurite, sodalite, quartz crystal, sapphire, tourmaline, lapis lazuli, and indicolite

Healing exercises:

Yoga, particularly child's pose or other forward-leaning poses

Eye exercises

CHAPTER 10: HEALING THE SEVENTH CHAKRA

The seventh, crown or Sahasrara, chakra is located at the very top of the head, above the line of the spine and where the crown touches air. It is known as the 'crowning chakra' not only because it sits atop the body but also because it helps to unify all of the body and the other chakras together and you into one spiritual being.

The crown chakra is known as the spiritual chakra, or the point where the spiritual realms open up for you, where enlightenment is possible, as well as the higher realms of being. By developing this chakra, it may be possible to find spiritual liberation, to interact with other spiritual beings, and as to develop our mystical experiences. This chakra is the essential component for all religions and beliefs and links us to our sense of idealism.

Physically, the crown chakra is also associated with our brain, our cerebrum, our cerebral cortex, and our central nervous system. It regulates the pineal and the pituitary glands as well as all of the hormones associated with them. When it is balanced, we have learned to transcend the ego, to become self-sufficient emotionally as well as intellectually, and to be filled with confidence.

If unbalanced, then the crown chakra can lead to feelings of worry, anxiety, confidence problems, and apathy. This may manifest physically as headaches, worry, anxiety, or even immune disorders.

When healing the seventh chakra, it is essential that greater attention is paid to the preceding chakras as well and not just to the crown itself. As the crowning and regulating chakra, it is wise to start at the bottom of the chakra system and work ones way up towards the crown, briefly stopping and aligning all of the previous chakras until we reach the top. In this way, we can stabilize the crown at its best and most productive, as a regulator and controller of the entire subtle body.

Related incense: Gotu kola or lotus

Related herbs: Nutmeg and gotu kola

Related aromatherapy: Clove, peppermint, and cinnamon

Associated glandular system: Pineal glands

Musical note: B

Chakra sound: Ohm

Element: Divine light, fire, and thought

Crystals: Sugilite, amethyst, purple fluorite, quartz, diamond, selenite, and alexandrite.

Color: Violet or divine white

Healing exercises:

Meditation

Running, jogging, and any other cardio system

THE CHAKRA CODE CONCLUSION

Thank you again for purchasing this book!

I hope this book was able to help you to balance your chakras naturally, instantly, and safely!

The next step is to start mapping your own chakra system out by using the techniques described inside to diagnose and douse each chakra. This will inform you immediately whether any chakra is currently out of line or imbalanced! After that, you can start to take the steps mentioned to associate each chakra with its elements, foods, and crystals, working to bring it back into balance naturally!

Finally, if you enjoyed this book, please take the time to share your thoughts and post a review on Amazon. It'd be greatly appreciated!

May The Energy Be With You,

Daniel Amos

Introduction

I want to thank you and congratulate you for purchasing the book, Kundalini Uncovered!

This book contains proven steps and strategies on how to awaken your inner potential using the power of the *Kundalini*, inherent in all human beings! This special force will help you to become healthier and more confident and creative and realize spiritual growth!

Over the course of this book, you will become acquainted with what Kundalini actually is and what it does to your body and mind. After this, you are provided with a range of proven strategies for igniting your own serpent power, from breathing techniques, visualizations, dancing, and more. Along the way, you will be given tips, hints, and step-by-step advice on how to utilize this ancient form of spiritual awakening and healing, in a totally demystifying, safe, and natural way.

Thanks again for purchasing this book, and I hope you enjoy it!

CHAPTER 1: KUNDALINI UNCOVERED

The Kundalini, otherwise called 'serpent energy,' is a natural source of energy that exists within everyone's body, usually kept in a dormant state until activated. It activates spontaneously in certain situations and, like other automatic physical responses, can be experienced as extreme, slight, or anywhere in between. Most people do not experience 'full' Kundalini during their life spans and don't even know that this power exists! However, as this is a natural energy response of the body and the mind, we can train our senses and our body to initiate Kundalini and also change the quality of the Kundalini 'awakening.'

Kundalini at a Glance

A sudden surge of intense energy and emotion from the base of the spine, the base chakra right up to the top of the head.

It affects your whole body; you feel it tingling your nervous, endocrine, and hormonal systems.

Some people experience great pleasure and muscle spasms, followed by deep bliss.

The Kundalini energy 'ignites' your chakras and your meridians, literally cleaning your subtle body of all impurities.

But How Does Kundalini Work? The Subtle Body

The subtle body is a concept that originated in Tantric Buddhist practice and can be found echoed throughout the Far East in the schools of Ayurveda, Chinese medicine, Reiki, yoga, and Tantra. It is a concept that does not rely upon any religious belief, but rather is an understanding of how our bodies and minds work.

The subtle body is the energetic field that exists within and all around us. In fact, everything that you can see, feel, hear, or even think is powered by this invisible energy variously called *chi, qi,* or *prana.* Modern-day science would call it the same as subatomic energy, which does not 'belong' to any particular object, but is loosely associated with certain molecular groupings. These subatomic energy waves interact, react, and transform each other in a never-ending dance of energy that is transmitted from the nuclear fusion deep within stars and radiates out across the universe.

The subtle body, therefore, is a way of understanding how to relate to that cosmic energy that makes up our bodies, our emotions, the world around us, and our entire notion of who we are. It refers to our personal 'sea' of energy that is generated by what we eat, how we feel, and what we are doing with our bodies. If we feel sad, then our subtle body diminishes, our immune system goes down, and we physically start to feel anxious, sick, and unwell. On the other hand, if we are happy, then our subtle body grows and we feel expansive, joyous, healthy, and confident.

The way the Kundalini works is that it operates between those two levels of the subtle and the physical. Actual physical activity such as yoga, dancing, and even sex can awaken the Kundalini, as well as supposedly spiritual activities such as meditation, visualization, and devotion. When we perform the right technique, then we awaken this automatic response that sends energy sizzling through our physical and our subtle bodies, unifying them and restoring them to their proper balance.

The Story of Kundalini

Because of this unique ability that Kundalini has to unify the spiritual and the physical, it sometimes has been called legendary or dismissed as even mythical. Other teachers warn caution and counsel against trying to awaken it too early.

It is only in Hatha yoga that the practice of Kundalini has been kept alive and brought through the years, and even today, it is yoga that regularly teaches people how to use and work with this powerful source.

Because of the unique properties of Kundalini, it is regarded as a spiritual and as a physical experience. This is because no one can guess when the Kundalini awakening will happen, they can only prepare for it. By taking the steps and performing the techniques demonstrated in this manual, we can show you how to prepare and bring on the Kundalini force within you. The Kundalini awakening itself will bring you an emotional awakening as well, as you find that your spiritual self is filled with powerful feelings. It is said that the awakening of the Kundalini force is the first step to enlightenment!

CHAPTER 2: THE KUNDALINI PROCESS

The Kundalini awakening is often described not just as a one-off event, but as a process that your whole body goes through. Just like any engagement with a sport, artistic endeavor, or serious work, you will find that the Kundalini impulse happens in smaller ways, randomly, and then later on, it reoccurs as you grow more proficient.

For many, this experience can be troubling or even upsetting, but for all, it can prove beneficial. There are a myriad of terms used to describe the Kundalini awakening, and generally, everyone agrees that you can experience it to a lesser or a greater extent often, throughout your life. Through the course of this guide, I will use the term 'full awakening' to indicate a Kundalini experience that is whole body and results in a deep spiritual experience at the same time. You may find that you experience this 'full awakening' or that you experience it in lesser degrees.

Many practitioners talk of feeling the surges of revitalizing and refreshing energy shoot up through the spin and rising feelings of joy, enthusiasm, and peace. Sometimes, you may experience this 'uncoiling' and 'rising' alone without the full-blown 'explosion' of spiritual ecstasy. Know that this is normal and a very good sign of progress! It shows that you have opened the Kundalini channels inside your body and that there is even now a rising energy using those channels.

Symptoms of Kundalini

Sometimes known as Kundalini syndrome, there are a number of symptoms that you can familiarize yourself with which will go some way to help you to acclimatize to the experience of Kundalini awakening. For some, this awakening can be a confusing or even a scary experience, especially if they have associated problems with their third eye chakra as well (see future guidebooks from this publisher).

The reason why some people experience negative symptoms is because they may not be properly grounded or not ready for the full awakening. It is advisable at this instant to return to healthy living and an honest, open attitude and to ground yourself in other Kundalini techniques, such as long deep breathing.

Positive Symptoms of Kundalini Include the Following:

The instantaneous healing of physical and emotional issues

The increased ability to achieve ever deeper meditative states

A general raised spiritual awareness, including an awareness of others, karma, and spiritual law

A profound sense of interconnectedness with God, nature, and your fellow humanity

The ability to heal other people by hand and sight or even to diagnose problems in others

Increased confidence, mental poise, and grace

Some Negative Symptoms of Kundalini Syndrome Include the Following:

Confusion or 'brain fog'

Intense emotions or mood swings

Sudden cramps or spasms

Pressure headaches

Uncontrollable feelings of energy rising up through the spine

How to Avoid a 'Bad Trip'

The most fundamental way to avoid the negative experiences associated with the Kundalini awakening is to remember that this is an all-body process, not a singular event. When you become much more comfortable with the science behind Kundalini, and the feelings that Kundalini can generate inside your body, you will begin to see that the Kundalini process is almost always, constantly ongoing.

Every time we exercise, we are using certain physical muscles to perform a task, and the task gets easier. The same is true of the Kundalini techniques – the more you meditate, the more open and confident and aware you become to these subtle energies. The more you learn your breathing techniques, the more you learn how to enter into and out of different states of consciousness and contribute to your good health and mental well-being.

Every time that you experience a Kundalini 'rise,' you will be taken a little further along the process of awakening towards full spiritual ecstasy. Quite simply – the more you do it, the better at it you get!

CHAPTER 3: THE KUNDALINI BREATH TECHNIQUE

Considered to be the 'easiest' or at least, the most straightforward way to ignite the Kundalini is to start by developing a successful breathing meditation. These exercises help you to regulate the flow of energy coming into and out of your body called *prana*. It is a technique perfected in the discipline of yoga, particularly Hatha yoga.

How to Start Learning Breathing Techniques

To start with, it is important not to already be suffering from any respiratory conditions, blood pressure problems, or otherwise serious conditions that will affect your ability to breathe continuously and in a directed manner.

It is best to not be a smoker or heavy drinker.

All techniques should begin from a comfortable seated position, in an ergonomic or a straight-backed chair, with support for the lower back. You should at all times feel comfortable, rested, and relaxed.

Learning How to Control Your Breath

It is a sad fact that most of us do not actually know how to breathe properly. We are taught to only take shallow breaths as if we are afraid of breathing too much or too deeply. It is worth reminding ourselves that breath itself is the source of life for our body. So breathe deep and feel nourished!

The first steps to controlling your breathing are to gently count a rhythm into your breathing, and a good place to start is to a count of four.

Breath in slowly, counting 1, 2, 3, 4 seconds.

Aim to fill your whole chest steadily with air.

At the end of the fourth, when you think that you cannot take any more, just take a tiny sip more.

Hold peacefully for the same count of four.

Exhale at a steady rate to another count of four, and at the end of that, when you think that you have exhaled all of your air out, huff just a little more.

As you develop this technique, you will become amazed at just how much air there is contained within four simple seconds! In time, and after weeks of this practice, you may be able to extend your count to five, and to six. Remember to try and keep your awareness light and gentle.

Do not try to force the breath, either on the in, hold, or out.

Try to find that brief moment between the breathing in and the hold and the hold and the out and that moment of stillness that exists in the tranquil center between action and non-action.

Moving the Breath

Learn how to move the feeling of the breath around your body during your mastery of the breath. In this way, you will begin to learn how to bring the breath up from your base chakra, right down at the bottom of your spine, and bring it up to the crown chakra. This is the essential process of activating the Kundalini.

First, during your practice, imagine when you breathe in that you are breathing in past your lips, mouth, and lungs and deep into your stomach, your abdomen, and past that into your base. You will feel that the breath has taken on the characteristics of heaviness and deepness.

When you breathe out, imagine it drawing up and out from the deepest parts of you, up and out – taking with it any impurities, worries, or anxieties. You will notice that you feel lighter, happier, and somehow 'brighter.' After you are experienced with this type of breathing, try to learn how to move your breath through your limbs, the extremities, and the top of your head. You can imagine the breath becoming lighter and more dynamic, and you may start to experience different sensations of the breath itself. Again, when you breathe out, do so fully and completely.

The Three Breath Techniques: Long Deep Breathing, Breath of Fire, and Alternate Nostril Breathing

When you have been practicing the above technique for a few weeks and have since become much more acquainted with your own breathing, you will be ready to start investigating the three tried-and-true techniques to bring on a Kundalini awakening.

These are the long deep breathing (or breathing with your whole diaphragm), the fire breath (or quickly pushing air out of your body and raising energy at the same time), and finally the alternate nostril breathing technique, (where you stimulate the different currents of the subtle body by bringing the air up and down your spine, igniting the Kundalini force).

It is important at all times to start from a relaxed position and in an alert and attentive state. If at times you start to feel dizzy, nauseous, or sick at any time, then of course it may be a sign for you to stop. You may suddenly find yourself experiencing Kundalini while performing these exercises, but you will almost certainly be forewarned by a sense of growing tension and energy rising up through the muscles of your body and your mind. It is important to have a good general acquaintance with all three of these techniques before you begin.

Technique 1: Long Deep Breathing

Long deep breathing is usually the first technique that Hatha yoga practitioners master, because it teaches you how to utilize the whole diaphragm in breathing.

Begin by sitting cross-legged, in full lotus position, or lying completely flat on the floor (otherwise known as corpse pose).

If sitting, breathe slowly in for a long moment, with hands on knees. Slightly lean forward and sit upright so that you can feel your diaphragm naturally expand.

When your lungs are completely filled, hold the breath lightly for a moment, before breathing out slowly, naturally letting your body empty out completely.

After some practice, it will start to feel as though your body is a complete balloon which is filling with air, before emptying again.

Technique 2: Breath of Fire (or Agni-Prasana)

The breath of fire is very different to long deep breathing; as with this exercise, you learn to expel air very forcefully through your abdominal contractions. It is taught as an advanced skill to purify and cleanse the subtle body, and it a quick way to energize yourself.

Start by performing the long deep breathing, feel it naturally flow into you, and expand your diaphragm.

After a few moments of this, gradually shift your awareness to the outward breath. You will notice that there is a pressure that the breath feels to expel itself out of the body and an immediate need to fill the lungs once more once empty.

Gently, and still in a meditative frame of mind, take your hands and place them on your abdomen and feel the rise and fall of your breath.

On your next outward breath, apply a little pressure to the breath from your abdomen, contracting as you exhale. You will notice that the breath empties much faster and forcefully.

Allow the inward breath to immediately refill as per normal.

On the next outward breath, again contract with the abdomen to speed the exhale.

This process should continue until you start to feel a bellows - like rhythm take over. Eventually, your outward breath should naturally become forceful that it makes a semipowerful 'Huh!' sound all of its own.

Try not to 'control' or direct this outward breath, but do so through the abdominal contractions.

Maintain this breath of fire for a few minutes.

The breath of fire charges the lower chakras and awakens them to release energy in a much more forceful way. After a few days and weeks of practicing this type of exercise, you will start to feel yourself becoming fuller and brighter, and your mental space will take on a 'clear' and expansive feeling.

Technique 3: Alternative Nostril Breathing

This is an advanced pranayama technique, taught in Hatha yoga and in some schools of Hinduism and Buddhism. It is used to charge and purify the different channels (or meridians) of the subtle body. Because of its cyclical nature, it actually allows the two sides of your body to interact to a much greater degree and encourages different states of consciousness.

Start by performing long deep breathing, until you feel relaxed, alert, and composed.

When you are ready, raise one hand, palm facing inwards towards your face. Rest one thumb against one side of your nose, closing the nostril, with the forefinger on the other side.

Breathe slowly in through the one open nostril and hold for a brief second. Concentrate on that still moment between breaths and exhale through the same nostril.

When you are ready to take your next breath, open the nostril by releasing your thumb and close off the alternate nostril with your forefinger. Breathe in through the alternate nostril in the same manner, hold for a moment, and then exhale through the open nostril.

Every time you go through a breathe in and exhale, you then alternate to breathe in and exhale through the alternate nostril, closing off the previous. Continue this for a short amount of time, until you start to feel tired.

You will soon start to feel a rising tension in your body, a 'charging' of your physical body and your mental mind state. You should feel this calming and energizing your mind-set and outlook and will immediately start to feel healthier and more confident!

CHAPTER 4: THE SHAKING MEDITATION

Another simple way to start to release your inner Kundalini energy is to simply 'shake it out'! Whereas the other techniques focus on preparing you for Kundalini awakening, the shaking method tried to activate your chakras in a much more fun and natural way, again using the principle synthesis of mind and body.

Tips

The shaking method is best performed at the end of the day, although at the very beginning of that day as well can be beneficial.

Whether you achieve full Kundalini awakening or not, the effect will be to start to break down ones inhibitions, prejudices, and 'rocklike' ego.

Some people like to use a long piece of regular, repetitive, and rhythmic music such as drumming, trance and dance music, or classical.

The Shaking Meditation

First Stage: Let your body dance and shake for 15mins, feeling your muscles relax and your energies flow from your feet upwards.

Second Stage: Allow yourself to free expression dance for 15mins, anyway that you want, using large and languid movements, and move around the space that you are occupying.

Third Stage: Close your eyes and be still for fifteen minutes, witnessing and observing your emotions, how you feel, and how your body is feeling.

Fourth Stage: Keeping your eyes completely closed, lie on the floor, and be completely still.

You may find that the Kundalini awakening happens during one of the active periods or, suddenly, rising up through the inactive 'silent' periods. Either will work to heal your body and to bring your subtle body energies back into alignment.

CHAPTER 5: THE KUNDALINI YOGA

Considered by many to be the purest form of Kundalini activation, the aim of Kundalini yoga is to awaken the Kundalini force just by a combination of gestures and meditation. This not only serves to prepare the mind for Kundalini awakening but also helps the individual to fully appreciate the more spiritual gifts that Kundalini can offer.

Tips

It is best, before you begin with this meditation, to be knowledgeable of meditation and relaxation techniques, as this will help you get into the right frame of mind and bodily position.

This meditation is best performed in full lotus, although half lotus or squatting on the floor (as long as your back can be straightened) is also acceptable.

Steps in Kundalini Yoga

Step 1:

Start by squatting or resting in a cross-legged or lotus position. Take a few deep breaths to prepare and cleanse your body.

Mentally allow your thoughts to settle and your worries to disappear.

When you feel calm and relaxed, you may begin.

Visualize the Earth below you as a giant circle and a star shining below you, inside of the Earth. Silently or just under your breath, say 'Earth' over and over as a mantra. Visualize the Earth below you filling with the light of the star, becoming bright and joyful and alive with energy. Rub the ground with your feet, feeling that energy comes flooding upwards.

Step 2:

Visualize a bright sun in the sky, flooding down light into you, your body, and the earth below.

Silently, or just under your breath, repeat the word 'sun' as a blessing and as a mantra, feeling the sun's energy filling you with light and health.

Rub your feet and feel the sun's energy crackle into them.

Step 3:

Visualize the star ascending up, through the earth and into your body. Feel yourself bathed in its light and healing your body, energizing you as it grows.

Silently or just under the breath, repeat the word 'body' as a mantra.

Visualize yourself being wrapped in healing, calm light.

Step 4:

'Clean' your body with the light of the star sequentially as it rises, washing away all impurities. Visualize the star's light rushing through and around your extremities, your limbs, your bones and organs, your torso and body, and your neck and head.

Silently or just under the breath, repeat the word 'light' as a mantra.

Step 5:

Raise both hands outwards from the elbows, palms upwards in the symbol of a universal blessing, and send that light out to another soul. Repeat the mantra that 'I bless (insert name), may all beings be happy, and may all beings be healed.'

Step 6:

Bring your hands to your belly and abdomen, and tense the muscles in your pelvis, abdomen, and chest.

Relax, and then contract once more. Breathe deeply and repeat the universal mantra of peace 'Om Shanti.'

Step 7:

In the final stage, return yourself to a calm meditation position, and focus on the line of energy that is in the middle of your spine and the core of your being. This is the Kundalini channel. You may feel it energized, throbbing, or even crackling with energy. Stay with that channel and that awareness until you naturally come out of meditation.

CHAPTER 6: SEX AND KUNDALINI

Obviously, no discussion on Kundalini would be complete without sex. In certain rare Tantric schools, sexual activity is indeed used to achieve states of divine consciousness, and in general, the awakening of the Kundalini is often likened to a form of sexual orgasm. Many of the symptoms are the same, such as hot flushes, the tension and concentration of energy in the base chakra and sexual organs, and then the release of energy upwards through the body.

By using the sexual impulse, it is possible to simulate Kundalini and even to bring on full Kundalini by allowing sexual activity to open up the Kundalini channel but then delaying the orgasm before the point of climax. By performing this repeatedly, the resulting tension is transferred spiritually, in an experience of divine ecstasy that effectively destroys the ego.

This same awareness of the loss of ego occurs naturally during sex, a fact that has led sex itself to be called in French as *la petite mort*, or the 'little death.' However, that moment of egolessness is often brief and fleeting, and soon, the ego mind starts to build itself up once again. The Kundalini process, on the other hand, leads to a much greater change in your spiritual nature, reducing the energies that make up the ego rather than temporarily delaying them.

The key difference between Kundalini energy and pure sexual activity is that Kundalini researchers are performing these actions constantly and deliberately delaying climax to reach a spiritual state. It is not merely about two people performing an act, but about overcoming duality and achieving oneness, or the divine.

The same effect can be replicated through enforced celibacy and by transmitting that sexual energy through the breathing techniques into a Kundalini awakening. Always be careful however that you are not using the Kundalini force as a tool just to hide sexual hang-ups or problems!

KUNDALINI UNCOVERED CONCLUSION

Thank you again for purchasing this book!

I hope this book was able to help you to *uncover Kundalini* and to experience greater states of healthiness, confidence, and spiritual balance in your life.

The next step is to start practicing control over your breath and to choose one of the techniques described in this book and start practicing!

Finally, if you enjoyed this book, please take the time to share your thoughts and post a review on Amazon. It'd be greatly appreciated!

May The Energy Be With You!

Daniel Amos

REIKI
Relax, De-Stress and Instantly Heal Your Body with This
Natural Energy Super Drug

Introduction

I want to thank you and congratulate you for purchasing the book, *Reiki!*

This book contains proven steps and strategies on how to use the power of *Reiki* to instantly heal, de-stress and repair your mind and body, returning it to its natural state of balance.

Through the next few chapters we will be taking a look at what Reiki is, and how you can use it to help you for your own personal development as well as for others. You may start to find, as you become more familiar with the techniques within this book, that people start turning to you for advice or help. This actually means that you doing your job well, and is all a part of the healer's journey.

Thanks again for purchasing this book, I hope you enjoy it!

CHAPTER 1: WHAT IS REIKI?

Reiki is an ancient form of natural energy medicine originally developed in Japan by a Buddhist monk named Mikao Usui, who was the first to put down on paper the meditative practices that he used to heal people.

The word Reiki itself is actually made up of two Japanese words – Rei and Ki, which do not have an exact translation in the English language, but can be approximately translated as Universal Energy and Personal Direction. Together, these words have a variety of subtle meanings, but are generally understood as linking the Universal Energy to your own, personal energy.

What it refers to, is the practice of attuning and cleaning your Ki or Chi, which is the divine energy that flows through all things.

Ki: The Universal Energy

Central to our understanding of Reiki is the belief in Ki, or universal, divine energy. Ki is found in all things, every rock, plant, vegetable, table, you, me and star. It is more present in living things, and 'accumulates' in living things as they take in available energy of what is around them. Quite simply, you get energy from food, the sun, your relationships and environment, the things that you see, read, and drink. All of these sources affect who you are and how you feel. We can see a belief in Ki that stretches right across the world, from the Chi of China, Prana of India, Ti for the Hawaiians as well as being called the bioplasma, orgone or odic force.

It is essential to understand that our Ki is always in flux, we are always experiencing either greater or lesser 'surges' of Ki depending upon our actions, and this will dictate our health. Ki, the universal energy is also called the *animating* energy that dictates how healthy, light and *alive* we feel. This is one of the prime reasons it is also linked with *light, light-working* or *colour therapy*.

Ki Blockages

Unfortunately for us, in today's hectic modern world we often cannot get the right amount or quality of Ki to feel as alive, rested and joyful as we should. There are some well-known symptoms of having a low or poor quality Ki:

Do you feel tired most of the time, achey?

Low moods or often irritable?

Do you suffer from constant low-grade, chronic illnesses or have a low immune system?

Do you often feel heavy, slothful and unhappy?

Do you feel restless, fidgety and anxious, as if you cannot settle or relax?

These are all symptoms of underlying Ki problem, which has to be addressed immediately if you do not wish to see it develop into something more serious!

If you have bad quality and low levels of Ki, then this means that the divine life force – the *animating* energy of the universe is having a hard time flowing through you. This is because of Ki blockages, which can take the form of trauma's, negative life experiences, unhealthy addictions or mental habits. The practice of Reiki seeks to clear those blockages, by allowing the universal, divine energy to flow through your body clear and strong!

Mind & Body Unity

An essential reason for how Reiki works is that it relies upon the fact that the mind and body are not separate, but are in fact one thing. In Western science and spirituality, it has always been taught (mostly because of Descartes) that the mind and body are two separate and distinct entities, making it difficult to see how they could even interact, let alone guide each other. However, the Eastern perspective makes more sense: it is obvious that when we are tired or that our body is run down then our mind is also affected. How many times have we been irritable and said the wrong thing after a long day at work?

Buddhists like Mikao Usui, our founder of Reiki have long talked about the unity of mind and body, stating that it is our mind that creates our actions, which create our Karma (or fortunes). Usui took this idea one step further, discovering the fact that our mind extends out just from the dome of our heads. Our good and bad emotions create for us our fortunes, by allowing us to interact joyfully and confidently with the world, or by lodging in our body and our environment if negative. How many times have you heard the phrase, sick with worry? Or have heard of people suffering nervous headaches, stomach aches because of stress and anxiety? In reality, we all know that our negative emotions can cause drastic changes in our physical body, even making us sick!

Whilst Reiki can 'clear' most of the negative, heavy Ki that accumulates in the body, what causes more of a problem are our subconscious negative thoughts and feelings. These are often negative reinforcements that we may have been carrying since childhood, such as that we are ugly, or stupid, or unsuccessful. Having these low grade negative reinforcements subtly changes the energy that we allow ourselves, and colours all of our thoughts and feelings.

Bad personal views, for instance, may encourage us to not look after our body, to eat poorly, to not exercise. They may stop us from seeing positive opportunities and relationships right in front of us.

How Reiki Can Help

The supreme value of Reiki is the fundamental concept that it is guided by divine power – remember the two words that made up the term? You are free to interpret this divine power as God, or to call it Universal Energy. Other Reiki practitioners I know interpret it as 'the way that the Universe wants to operate' as a healthy, functioning, growing energy. Remember that every apparently mindless seed germinates with enthusiasm for life, opportunity and animation.

When you learn how to practice Reiki, you are calling upon this divine energy to descend into your body and your life, clearing the negative blockages and to *restore the natural balance to your body*. This last bit is essential. You are asking the energy to bring the body back to its natural state of light, clear, joyful and enthusiasm.

Remember too, that Reiki works on a mental as well as a physical level. It acts on your thoughts and beliefs as much as it does on any physical conditions that you may have, because of the unity of mind and body principle.

How Do I Learn Reiki?

Unlike other programmes of spiritual excellence, Reiki does not ask you to spend years studying comparative religions, or to invest large amounts of money. As Reiki is all about connecting with the universal, divine energy it is necessarily free-to-use, at point of need.

Instead, knowledge of Reiki can be 'transmitted' to you through Reiki masters in stages called 'attunements'. There are many different Reiki schools out there, each of which offer to attune you to your desired level, some can perform this act remotely, through online sources, whilst often you will find in your local areas work groups called Reiki Circles that can offer to transmit Reiki practice to you. Some groups or Grandmasters will perform this service – which is a non-touch, non-invasive, silent spreading of energy, for free, whilst others will charge.

There three 'Grades' to traditional Reiki, first or 'beginner' grade, second (which encourages you to spread your wisdom and heal others, and the final third 'Grandmaster' grade which confers the ability to transmit the knowledge of Reiki to others.

If you find all this talk of attunements and Grandmasters daunting – don't worry! Because, you will be glad to hear, that you do not need to go through any daunting training process and, indeed, many practitioners pick up the principles simply by following the practice of Reiki meditation. All that it takes for you to start being able to use the power of Reiki to heal and relax yourself, is to start by practising the techniques in the Chapter 2.

Things to Remember:

Reiki can be learned at any age.

Reiki can be learned by anyone – it is a natural human ability.

Reiki does not use any form of physical therapy.

Reiki does not require you to use any drugs, remedies, medicines or pills.

Reiki can work with almost any religion or spiritual belief systems that you already have.

Reiki does not ask you to convert or to believe any particular religion or system. Actually, many practitioners have noted that it doesn't matter whether you believe in *it* or not!

CHAPTER 2: HEALING YOURSELF

To begin using Reiki, you must familiarize yourself with three things: the **Guiding Reiki Principles**, **Meditation**, and the **Gassho Technique**. These three things are, ultimately all that you need to heal your body and de-stress your life. However, there are extra and more advanced Reiki techniques later on in this book for you develop your spiritual skills.

The Guiding Reiki Principles.

These three principles are the original tenets of Reiki, as outlined first by Mikao Usui almost a hundred years ago. He stated that these fundamental principles allow the practitioner of Reiki to become a clear conduit for divine, universal energy, and that by paying heed to them they will allow you to do the same.

1. *Just for today, I will not anger.*

2. *Just for today, I will not worry and will be filled with gratitude.*

3. *Just for today, I will devote myself to this work, and will be kind to others.*

You can follow these principles as stringently or as loosely as you wish, but the purer your intentions are and the more optimistic and loving your outlook it, the more benefit you are sure to get out of your Reiki practice.

The idea behind following the Reiki principles is that they ground your Reiki practice in positive energy, and start clearing you of the negative or heavy Ki by encouraging positive, hopeful and joyful emotions. As we all know, anger and worry are very destructive emotions either to feel or to carry around with us, causing further blockages within our own bodies. This is why it is important to try to observe Usui's three principles to help you to use this ancient and powerful energy.

Meditation

The science of meditation isn't just sitting quietly in a corner and looking at your navel. That is actually the smallest part of it! Meditation, as a form of relaxation encompasses contemplation, tranquility, insight and creative visualization; all of which are tools which you use to clear and focus your mind.

Reiki itself can be called a form of meditation, as it generates a meditative state through which the universal energy flows. Meditation also develops your awareness and skill with Reiki energy, and so is a good practice to take up!

The Health Benefits of Meditation

Scientific studies performed on experienced meditators have found that those in a meditative state encourage the brains to emit more Alpha waves, associated with periods of concentration and deep sleep. Alpha Waves are thought to be used by the brain to process large amounts of information as well as to re-order and to 'heal' itself!

But not only that, meditation also holds remarkable benefits for your body as well. Similar studies have shown how meditators benefit from lower blood pressure, a slower heart rate, as well as an increased oxygen-to blood ratio and more robust immune systems and fewer chronic illnesses! It is believed that Tibetan Monks who were also tested have shown remarkable abilities to slow down their own heart rate and decrease or increase their own body temperature!

Meditation allows us also to relax mentally, allowing our negative emotions to resolve themselves without having to resort to toxic pharmaceutical medicines or painful therapy.

Simple Reiki Meditation 1

Begin by sitting or lying down in a comfortable position. Make sure that, if lying down completely prone that it is not too late at night or that you are too sleepy. If in a chair, make sure that your lower back is supported.

You should feel comfortable but not slouching. Comfortable and alert.

Take a few deep breaths, and try to let go of all of your current worries and concerns. If you find that there is something currently obsessing or worrying you, hold it in your mind for just a moment, silently acknowledging it, and say, internally *'I know that you are there, but right now I am going to meditate'*. It is important to recognize what is on our minds, and to be able to let them go and turn to the task at hand.

Don't *try* to think of anything in particular, just allow your mind to settle into whatever rhythm it feels comfortable in. When you find that your thoughts are starting to run away on one issue or another, gently remind yourself that you are trying to meditate, acknowledge the thoughts and bring yourself back to a place of peace and quiet. The important thing, is not to *fight* your own mind, but to be gentle.

Your breathing should be steady and relaxed, not labored or forced.

As your mind clears you will start to feel calmer and more focused. If it helps, you can concentrate upon one thing – a candle or some soothing music, but you can just as easily keep your mind clear. The point of Reiki meditation is to be guiding the mind back to this state of calm and poised tranquility *'like a still pond, with hidden and deep depths'*.

When you feel calm and collected, imagine waves of radiant white light flowing down into you from above, over the crown of your head, and into your body. As the waves move through you, feel yourself growing calmer, clearer and more confident with every breath.

Mentally thank the universe for this gift, as gratitude is a very important spiritual practice.

Soon thereafter, you will start to feel tranquil and at peace. Enjoy this sensation – it is very healing, and works on your subconscious mind to ease any hidden anxieties or negative reinforcements that you may have.

When you feel collected, and ready to come out of your meditation, then take a few more breaths and prepare to re-engage with the world around you. Awaken gradually, first by opening your eyes, and then by breathing deeply. Finish by something physical, perhaps clapping your hands together or stamping your feet. Sometimes meditators feel 'distanced' from their bodies, so it is necessary for you to feel at home in your physical self once again. Try a glass of water and eating something.

When to Practice Your Reiki Meditation?

Really, there is no set or desirable time for you to practice meditation, other than *now!* Some people find meditation easier in the morning, before their day begins, or later on in the early evening, when their work day has ended. Others find these times to be their 'mental download' time, during which their brains are working overload! You will have to find a time, preferably once a day that feels comfortable to you to practice your Reiki Meditation.

Ideally you should be practicing for about 20 to 40 minutes a day, each day to get the most benefit, but remember that *any* time that you spend meditating will also help your familiarity with Reiki energy. Even if you only have ten minutes before work or during your lunch break, it is better to perform a 'mini meditation' than to not practice that day at all!

The Gassho Technique

The Gassho Technique is the founding practice of Reiki, described by Usui himself as all you really need in order to practice Reiki. By using your familiarity with Meditation and relaxation learned above you then apply this knowledge to generating the universal energy that will flow through you.

Start by sitting or standing in an alert but relaxed pose. You should feel physically comfortable, but not tired or 'heavy'.

Take a few deep and calming breaths, just the same as when you are about to start a Reiki Meditation. Allow your worries and anxieties to subside, recognizing them and allowing them to fade into the background.

When you feel ready, start by entering into a light meditative state, by visualizing the white, cleansing light fall down and fill you with love.

Bring up your hands as if in the traditional prayer position, and hold them just in front of your heart, palms facing each other but not quite touching.

Whilst in a calm, clear state imagine that positive energy of Universal love and light flowing down your arms, out from your heart chakra and into the space between your hands. After a while you will begin to feel a tingling sort of sensation between your palms. Some people claim to feel heat, light, or pressure.

Every time you breathe in, imagine that universal energy flowing into you. Every time you breathe out, imagine the air around your arms and the space between your hands filling with that energy. It is a calming, loving and peaceful energy.

Sit with your awareness of that energy, feeling it tingle along your palms and play over your hands.

When you are ready, start to send that energy towards your heart chakra (located just behind your solar plexus). You will feel your heart opening up in waves of gratitude, light and positivity, overflowing and filling your body with light, health and happiness.

Imagine that healing energy travelling around and filling your body, either by visualizing white light or green waves of energy. Everywhere that energy touches and fills, will be left feeling refreshed, relaxed and healthier. When you are experienced at Reiki you will be able to direct this energy at will.

When you are finished, or after about 10 – 20 minutes of healing, gradually return any residual energy back to your heart chakra and say a quiet thank you to the universe.

By practicing the Gassho Healing Technique every day, you will find yourself feeling lighter, healthier and a more open and relaxed individual. You are, quite literally aligning yourself with the life that you are meant to lead!

The Full Reiki Self-Treatment

When you feel that you are ready, after you are familiar with both Reiki Meditation and the Gassho Technique, you may feel comfortable offering yourself a full Reiki Self-treatment, which is the same basic treatment that you will eventually be performing for others in the final chapter.

As you develop as a Reiki master you will discover that there are as many ways to practice Reiki as there are Reiki practitioners! Some prefer to be lying down whilst others prefer to be seated. Some use colors or sound therapy, others like to chant or recite affirmations. You will find the system that best works for you by listening to the energy, and your heart. As you become more aware of your own marvelous capabilities, you will know what works and what doesn't!

Start by lying down in a comfortable position, with eyes closed. Try not to choose a time when you are likely to be too sleepy! Consider placing a pillow behind the head and under the lower back for comfort and also to make it easier to move your arms and elbows.

Engage in a light Gassho meditation, taking deep, cleansing breaths and allowing yourself to feel filled with light. Feel that energy pooling into the space between your hands.

Move your hands slowly down your body not actually touching the body) and hover for a few minutes over each of these locations:

The Crown of the Head

The Face

The Throat

The Upper Chest

Just under the Lowest Ribs

Over the Navel

The Lower Abdomen.

Each of these places outlined are the main energy centers of the body, and the places where your natural Ki 'puddles' or naturally collects.

Just as before with the Gassho Technique you feel light and radiance spreading from your hands, and you will also start to feel more relaxed and refreshed. If it helps you can also visualize the light moving down through the body in waves.

After a while, you may begin to notice that certain parts of the body that your hands are hovering over feel heat, cold or otherwise tingly. Depending upon your experience, these could be indicators of blockages or hidden subconscious negativities. Don't worry, these feelings are natural and you will know them instantly upon finding them. Some of the ways that Reiki practitioners describe Ki blockages are;

Sharp, almost uncomfortable tingling in their palms.

Sudden icy cold feelings, or sudden uncomfortable heat.

An inner sensation dread and low mood, localized around that body part.

A squirm of anxiety in your gut.

You will also feel, as soon as you start spreading that love into that area from the universal energy that those feelings begin to shift, loosen and that you start to feel lighter, happier and restored. This reaction is inevitable, as the positive, universal healing energy cannot be 'overcome' or blocked – it *is* the animating principle of the universe!

The practice of Reiki is, essentially the practice of encountering and removing these Ki blockages, and every time that you perform this full self-treatment, Reiki Meditation and the Gassho Technique you will be working on them in subtle, healing ways.

Some people also like to feel that energy moving down through the extremities of the arms and the legs as well, to finally feel as though the energy is fully 'washing-through'. However, do remember that the universal Ki energy is really a force in its own right, and that you are only its conduit. It is quite sufficient just to help it flow into your body in order for to take advantage of its healing properties!

CHAPTER 3: HEALING OTHERS

Using Reiki on Other People

Using Reiki to heal other people is actually to use Reiki as it was originally intended by its founder. He discovered that the universal energy of light and love was free, and was for the benefit of all living things. Using it to heal others is actually to use it for its original purpose.

When performed on other people Reiki is often performed in treatments, lasting between 20 – 40 minutes long, with the patient lying down and the Reiki practitioner channeling the energy through themselves and to the patient below.

The Reiki practitioner starts by asking their patient to take a few deep breaths and relax whilst they, too start to lightly meditate, and bring their hands to in front of their chest in the classic Gassho pose.

When they feel that tingle of energy and love, the practitioner moves from the top of the head down the body in slow movements just as if she were practicing on her own body, feeling where any blockages might be, and asking for the energy to pour into those places.

The patient usually has their eyes closed to help with their relaxation.

The Reiki practitioner may choose to put on some spiritual or calming music in the background. Often this helps to relax the patient, and gives their conscious mind something to interact with whilst their unconscious engages with the healing.

Whilst healing others you may find it necessary to return to places where you feel that there are significant blockages, and a variety of movements are encouraged to help direct the flow of energy.

Focused, hands over one spot position

Sweeping movements in the air above the blockage, down limbs etc.

Gentle 'pushing' or 'encouraging' hand movements above the affected area.

It is very important to visualize that area filling with love, light and healing as you perform this meditation. This mental 'blessing' will help you to fully engage with the practice.

The Reiki Circle/Reiki Share

Called the Mawashi Technique, the Reiki Circle is a way of spreading the power of Reiki energy through other people who also have an awareness of light working. It was first outlined by the discoverer of Reiki itself, who encouraged the students that he taught to practice this often. It is a way to heal each other and direct large quantities of Ki energy towards large healing projects.

Every person involved should have some awareness of healing, energy work or working with Reiki energy.

Everyone sits or stands comfortably in a circle, and lightly meditates using the Gassho technique.

After a few minutes, when the practitioners are ready, they all stretch out their arms to clasp each other's hands. The touch should feel electrifying and pure.

Imagine waves of the energy spreading out from your heart into those around you, just as others direct that energy in towards you. You will feel a sort of exponential 'doubling' of light energy, and some people have claimed to have seen light balls, sudden colors and deep feelings of bliss.

After about 5-15 minutes this energy can be returned each to their own heart chakra, or the group can decide to 'send' that energy to another source. Many Reiki Circles come together to perform Mawashi at times of great need, during disasters, or to aid someone who is ill. Imagine that energy being sent through the atmosphere to its target, illuminating their life and body with healing light and love!

Unexpected Benefits!

As this guide can only cover the basics of healing yourself with the universal energy of light and life that is Reiki, there are still many Techniques and mysteries out there for you to discover.

Some practitioners have developed ways to focus Reiki energy on specific ailments such Ear, Nose and Throat, the Spine, even chronic or acute illnesses by using a combination of special hand movements and visualizations.

What is true across the Reiki community is that it offers everyone in contact with it deep relaxation and psychological healing, allowing us to feel refreshed and lighter as a result.

You may start to discover numerous unexpected benefits from your practice, as your life begins to fall more into the rhythm of the universe. When you are following the Three Principles and actively healing your own Ki then you are living the life of the person you were meant to be, with access to far more possibilities than the normal person, weighed down with anxieties and unresolved issues.

Some Reiki practitioners talk about being able to diagnose illness just with a glance.

Being able to sense others emotions.

Other resort unexpected good fortune or premonitions warning them of possible ill.

All of these are signs that you are aligning yourself with universal energy, and that your unconscious is gradually picking up the subtle signals all around you about your friends, your environment and – the deepest mystery of all – yourself.

REIKI CONCLUSION

Thank you again for purchasing this book!

I hope this book was able to help you to discover the power of universal Reiki, to help you De-Stress and relax.

The next step is to follow the three practices outlined in Chapter 1, the Three Principles, Reiki Meditation and the Gassho Technique every day to start feeling the benefits!

Finally, if you enjoyed this book, please take the time to share your thoughts and post a review on Amazon. It'd be greatly appreciated!

May The Energy Be With You!

Daniel Amos
Afflatus Group LLC